ALOPECIA AREATA
NAVIGATING PATCHY HAIR LOSS AND FINDING HOPE

Dr. Mukesh Aggarwal

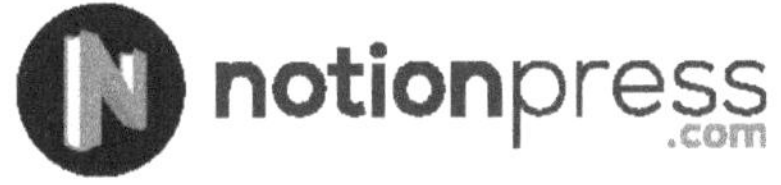

PREFACE

Dear Reader,

Welcome to a journey through the intricate landscape of alopecia areata – a condition that touches the lives of many, yet often remains misunderstood. As a Ayurveda Trichologist, my encounters with patients and their poignant narratives inspired the creation of this book.

The pages ahead aim to be a guiding light for those grappling with the uncertainties of alopecia areata. Through a blend of medical insights, personal stories, and holistic approaches, this book strives to illuminate the multifaceted dimensions of this condition.

Alopecia areata isn't just about hair loss; it's about resilience, emotional fortitude, and the unwavering spirit of those affected. In these chapters, I aspire to offer not just information but a sense of camaraderie and understanding.

Drawing from the collective experiences of patients, the expertise of medical professionals, and the strides made in research, this book endeavors to paint a comprehensive picture. From diagnosis to treatment options, emotional well-being to the promising horizon of future advancements, I aim to provide a compass for both individuals navigating this condition and those seeking a deeper understanding.

To the readers embarking on this exploration, may this book serve as a beacon of knowledge, empathy, and hope. Thank you for joining me on this journey to unravel the mysteries of alopecia areata.

Warm regards,
Dr. Mukesh Aggarwal

ACKNOWLEDGEMENTS

I am profoundly grateful to the individuals who made this book on Alopecia Areata possible. My heartfelt appreciation goes to the patients and their families who generously shared their experiences and stories, enriching the content and providing invaluable insights.

I extend my deepest gratitude to the medical professionals and researchers whose dedication and contributions have advanced our understanding and treatment of Alopecia Areata. Your commitment to this field is truly commendable.

I am indebted to my family for their unwavering support, understanding, and encouragement throughout this journey. Their love and patience have been the cornerstone of my work.

Lastly, I express my sincere thanks to the publishing team whose expertise and guidance have shaped this book into a resource aimed at offering hope and assistance to those affected by Alopecia Areata.

Dr. Mukesh Aggarwal

CONTENTS

INTRODUCTION

PURPOSE OF THE BOOK

The purpose of this book on alopecia areata is multifaceted, aiming to provide comprehensive support, information, and empowerment to individuals impacted by this condition.

The introduction sets the tone, highlighting the book's mission to offer guidance and hope to those navigating the challenges of patchy hair loss. It seeks to create a resource that informs and comforts readers dealing with alopecia areata, guiding them through various aspects of their journey.

Chapter 1 sets the foundation by defining alopecia areata, explaining its types, symptoms, prevalence, and potential causes. This section aims to educate readers, ensuring they understand the condition they're facing, reducing fear or uncertainty.

Moving into Chapter 2, the focus shifts to the emotional and psychological impact of alopecia areata. This section delves into coping strategies, the importance of support systems, and how relationships and social dynamics might be affected. Its purpose is to address the holistic impact on an individual's life beyond physical changes.

Chapter 3 delves into the medical perspective, equipping readers with knowledge about diagnosis, available treatments, ongoing research, and promising advancements. Its aim is to empower readers with information about medical interventions and to instill hope through the progress being made in the field.

Chapter 4 centers on lifestyle management and self-care. It aims to provide practical advice, including nutrition's role, haircare tips, and the impact of exercise and stress management. The purpose is to empower readers by offering tangible strategies to help manage their condition and overall well-being.

Chapter 5 shifts the focus to personal narratives and stories of resilience from individuals affected by alopecia areata. This section serves to inspire and create a sense of community, showcasing how others have navigated their journey and advocating for awareness and support.

Finally, Chapter 6 offers a glimpse into the future of alopecia areata research, highlighting breakthroughs and promising treatments on the horizon. Its purpose is to provide optimism and reinforce hope for advancements that could potentially change the landscape of managing this condition.

In essence, the book's purpose amalgamates information, support, empowerment, and hope. It aims to be a comprehensive guide that not only educates but also empathizes with and uplifts those impacted by alopecia areata, fostering a sense of community and resilience amidst their journey.

CHAPTER 1

WHAT IS ALOPECIA AREATA

DEFINITION OF ALOPECIA AREATA

Alopecia areata is a condition that causes hair loss in small, round patches on the scalp or other areas of the body. It's an autoimmune disease where the immune system mistakenly attacks hair follicles, leading to hair loss. The exact cause is not entirely understood, but genetics, environmental factors, and immune system abnormalities might play a role. This condition can vary widely in severity and can sometimes result in complete hair loss on the scalp (alopecia totalis) or the entire body (alopecia universalis).

TYPES:

Alopecia Areata (Patchy Hair Loss): Characterized by round patches of hair loss on the scalp or body.

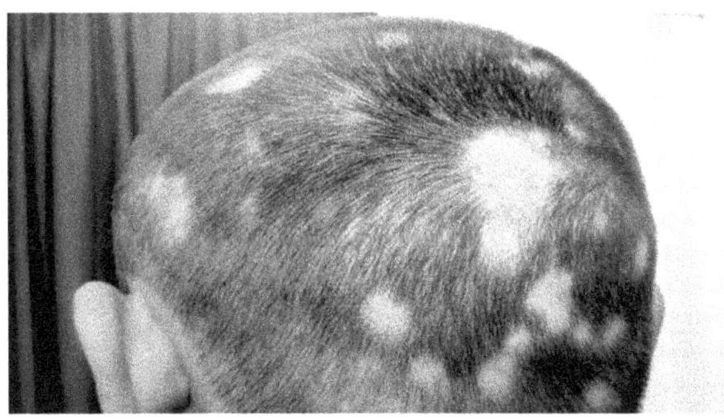

Alopecia Totalis: Complete loss of hair on the scalp.

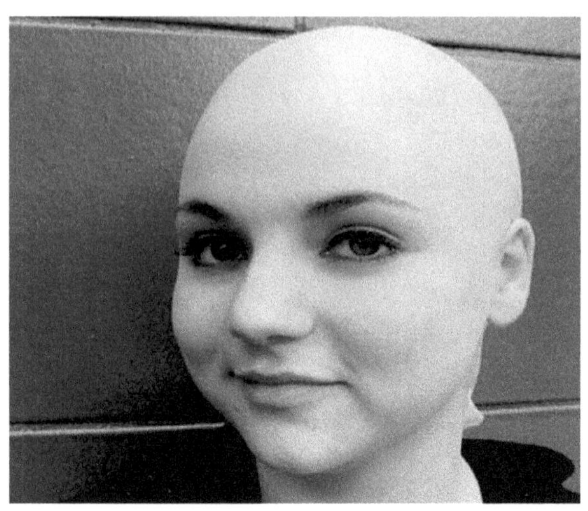

Alopecia Universalis: Total loss of hair on the entire body.

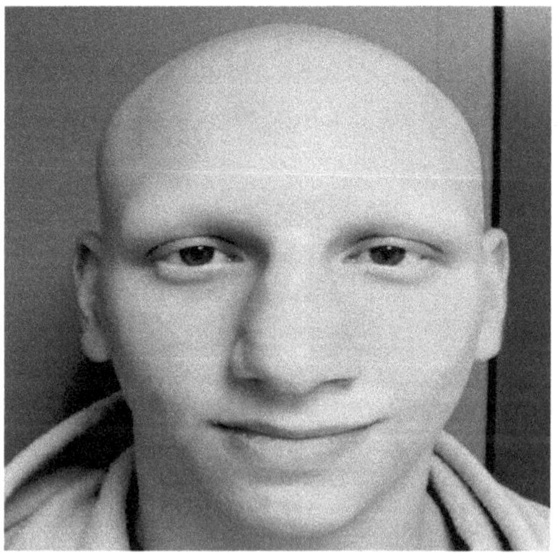

SYMPTOMS:

Sudden onset of hair loss in small, round patches.

Smooth, round bald patches on the scalp or other hair-bearing areas.

Sometimes, tingling or slight pain in the affected areas.

Nail abnormalities might accompany hair loss in some cases.

PREVALENCE:

Alopecia areata is relatively common, affecting about 2% of the population at some point in their lives.

It can occur at any age but often begins in childhood or early adulthood.

Both men and women are equally affected by this condition.

The symptoms and severity can vary greatly from person to person. Some may experience only one episode of hair loss, while others might have recurring instances or progress to more extensive baldness. Treatment approaches aim to stimulate hair regrowth and manage the condition's impact on an individual's life.

POSSIBLE CAUSES AND TRIGGERS

The exact cause of alopecia areata isn't fully understood, but it's believed to be a combination of genetic, environmental, and immune system factors. Several possible causes and triggers are associated with its onset and progression:

CAUSES:

Autoimmune Response: The immune system mistakenly attacks hair follicles, disrupting normal hair growth.

Genetics: Family history of autoimmune diseases or a genetic predisposition can increase the likelihood of developing alopecia areata.

Environmental Factors: Stress, trauma, infections, or other environmental triggers might play a role in initiating or exacerbating the condition.

TRIGGERS:

Stress: Emotional or physical stress can trigger or exacerbate episodes of hair loss.

Illness or Infections: Certain illnesses or infections might be linked to the onset of alopecia areata.

Hormonal Changes: Hormonal changes, particularly during pregnancy or with thyroid disorders, could be a trigger.

Allergens: Exposure to certain allergens or environmental triggers could contribute to the condition.

Identifying specific triggers for an individual can be challenging, as they can vary widely among people affected by alopecia areata. Managing stress and seeking medical advice for underlying health conditions might help in controlling or minimizing its impact.

LIVING WITH ALOPECIA AREATA

EMOTIONAL AND PSYCHOLOGICAL ASPECTS OF ALOPECIA AREATA

Alopecia areata, beyond its physical manifestation, deeply impacts individuals emotionally and psychologically. This autoimmune condition, resulting in hair loss, often triggers profound emotional distress due to its unpredictable nature and its impact on one's identity and self-esteem.

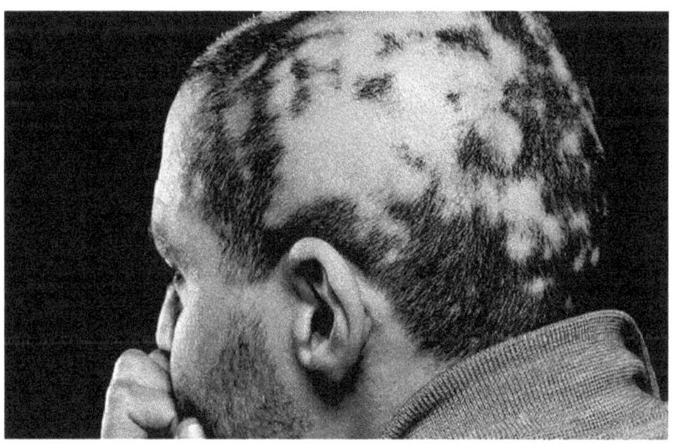

Firstly, the sudden and unpredictable nature of hair loss in alopecia areata can cause heightened emotional distress. The loss of hair, a fundamental part of one's appearance, challenges the sense of control individuals have over their bodies, leading to feelings of powerlessness and anxiety about the future. The uncertainty of whether the condition will progress or regress further adds to the emotional turmoil, causing individuals to constantly grapple with fear and apprehension.

Moreover, the societal perception of beauty and attractiveness tied to a full head of hair exacerbates the psychological impact of alopecia areata. The change in appearance can lead to a loss of self-confidence, affecting social interactions, relationships, and even professional opportunities. This alteration in self-perception might trigger feelings of isolation, depression, and low self-worth, especially in a culture that often associates hair with youthfulness and beauty.

Furthermore, the emotional toll of alopecia areata extends beyond the individual experiencing the condition. Family members and close friends might also grapple with their emotions, feeling helpless or distressed witnessing their loved one's struggle, further amplifying the psychological impact.

However, amidst these challenges, it's crucial to recognize the resilience individuals with alopecia areata often demonstrate. Many find strength in support groups, counseling, or therapies aimed at fostering self-acceptance and coping strategies. Additionally, raising awareness and fostering a more inclusive societal perception of beauty can significantly alleviate the emotional burden for those affected by this condition.

In conclusion, alopecia areata's emotional and psychological effects reach far beyond its physical manifestations. Understanding and addressing the emotional impact are crucial in supporting individuals dealing with this condition, promoting self-acceptance, and nurturing a more inclusive and empathetic society.

COPYING STRATEGIES AND SUPPORT SYSTEMS

Copying strategies and support systems are essential elements in navigating life's challenges, offering individuals tools and networks to manage difficulties effectively. These strategies encompass various techniques and mechanisms that aid in handling stress, adversity, and demanding situations.

One of the primary coping strategies involves problem-solving, wherein individuals actively tackle the issue at hand by identifying the problem, generating potential solutions, and implementing the most feasible one. This approach empowers individuals to take control of their circumstances, fostering a sense of efficacy and resilience.

Emotion-focused coping strategies, on the other hand, revolve around managing the emotional distress caused by a situation rather than directly addressing the issue itself. Techniques like mindfulness, relaxation exercises, and seeking emotional support aim to regulate emotions and reduce the impact of stress on mental well-being.

Another coping strategy involves seeking social support. This support network comprises friends, family, colleagues, or support groups, providing individuals with a sense of belonging, empathy, and advice. Sharing experiences and feelings within these networks often alleviates emotional burdens and helps individuals gain perspective on their situation.

Additionally, adopting a proactive approach by maintaining a healthy lifestyle through exercise, proper nutrition, and adequate sleep serves as a foundational coping strategy. Physical well-being significantly influences mental resilience, contributing to better stress management and overall coping abilities.

Moreover, professional support systems, such as therapy, counseling, or mental health services, play a pivotal role in providing specialized assistance tailored to individual needs. These services offer a safe space for individuals to explore their emotions, develop coping skills, and receive guidance from trained professionals.

In conclusion, coping strategies encompass a diverse range of techniques and support systems that individuals employ to manage life's challenges effectively. By utilizing problem-solving approaches, emotional regulation techniques, social support networks, healthy lifestyle habits, and professional assistance, individuals can navigate difficult situations with greater resilience and strength. Embracing these strategies fosters personal growth and equips individuals with the tools necessary to overcome adversities and thrive in various aspects of life.

RELATIONSHIPS AND SOCIAL DYNAMICS FOR ALOPECIA AREATA PATIENT

The experience of alopecia areata significantly influences relationships and social dynamics for those affected by the condition, impacting both personal connections and interactions within broader social circles.

At its core, alopecia areata can transform intimate relationships. Close partners, family members, and friends often play a crucial role in supporting individuals coping with the emotional and psychological challenges of hair loss. Understanding, empathy, and unwavering support from loved ones can alleviate the distress caused by the condition, fostering a sense of acceptance and resilience.

However, alopecia areata can also strain relationships, especially if individuals struggle to cope with the changes in appearance and the emotional toll it brings. Communication breakdowns or feelings of inadequacy might emerge, potentially challenging the bond between partners, family members, or friends. In such cases, open dialogue, education about the condition, and mutual support become pivotal in maintaining healthy relationships.

Social dynamics in broader circles can also be affected by alopecia areata. Social stigma or misconceptions surrounding hair loss can lead to uncomfortable interactions or societal pressures. Individuals might face judgment, discrimination, or insensitive remarks, impacting their confidence and willingness to engage in social settings.

Navigating professional environments can present additional challenges. The impact of alopecia areata on self-esteem and confidence might affect work dynamics, particularly if the individual feels self-conscious or experiences reduced self-assurance due to the condition.

Supportive work environments that foster inclusivity and understanding play a crucial role in helping individuals thrive despite the challenges posed by alopecia areata.

Despite these challenges, many individuals find strength within themselves and in the support systems around them. Support groups, online communities, and advocacy organizations provide platforms for sharing experiences, offering encouragement, and promoting awareness about alopecia areata. These networks serve as a source of solidarity, empowerment, and understanding, enabling individuals to navigate social situations more confidently.

In conclusion, alopecia areata profoundly influences relationships and social dynamics, both within intimate circles and broader social settings. While it can strain some relationships and trigger societal challenges, understanding, empathy, and education play critical roles in fostering acceptance and support. By nurturing supportive relationships, promoting awareness, and advocating for inclusivity, society can create a more empathetic and understanding environment for individuals affected by alopecia areata to thrive.

CHAPTER 3

DIAGNOSIS AND TREATMENT

DIAGNOSIS OF ALOPECIA AREATA

Alopecia areata, a dermatological condition, manifests as sudden hair loss, often in patches on the scalp or body. While the exact cause remains unclear, it's believed to stem from an autoimmune reaction targeting hair follicles. Diagnosing alopecia areata involves a comprehensive approach that considers clinical signs, medical history, and sometimes specific tests.

To diagnose alopecia areata, a dermatologist initially conducts a physical examination, inspecting the affected areas for characteristic hair loss patterns. Typically, the loss appears as smooth, round patches with no signs of inflammation or scarring. Patients might also report a rapid onset of hair shedding or noticing clumps of hair falling out.

An essential aspect of diagnosis involves discussing the patient's medical history, including familial predisposition to autoimmune diseases or previous occurrences of alopecia areata. Stressful events or illness might also be considered, as they can trigger or exacerbate the condition.

Sometimes, a dermatologist might perform a pull test to evaluate hair loss severity. This involves gently tugging on several strands of hair to observe the amount that comes out, aiding in assessing the stage and extent of the condition.

Additionally, in more complex cases or to rule out other potential causes of hair loss, a dermatologist may conduct a scalp biopsy. This procedure involves taking a small sample of the affected skin for microscopic examination, allowing for a closer evaluation of the hair follicles and surrounding tissue.

Furthermore, advanced diagnostic tools such as trichoscopy—an imaging technique allowing detailed examination of the scalp and hair follicles—can aid in confirming the diagnosis and monitoring the progression of alopecia areata.

In conclusion, diagnosing alopecia areata requires a combination of clinical observation, medical history assessment, and occasionally, supplementary tests. Collaborating with a dermatologist is essential for accurate identification and management of this condition, offering patients better understanding and suitable treatment options for their unique circumstances.

MEDICAL TREATMENT OF ALOPECIA AREATA

Treating alopecia areata involves various approaches aimed at managing the condition and promoting hair regrowth. While there isn't a definitive cure, several treatments aim to stimulate hair growth and reduce the autoimmune response targeting hair follicles.

Topical Treatments: Corticosteroids in the form of creams, ointments, or solutions applied directly to the affected areas can help reduce inflammation and encourage hair regrowth. Minoxidil, a topical solution commonly used for male and female pattern baldness, might also be prescribed to stimulate hair growth in some cases of alopecia areata.

Intralesional Corticosteroid Injections: Dermatologists may administer corticosteroid injections directly into the bald patches. This method is effective in suppressing the immune response and promoting hair regrowth.

Immunotherapy: This approach involves applying certain chemicals like diphencyprone (DPCP) or squaric acid dibutyl ester (SADBE) to the scalp, which aims to provoke an allergic reaction. This reaction shifts the immune response away from targeting hair follicles, potentially allowing hair regrowth.

Anthralin: This topical medication alters the skin's immune function and is applied to affected areas, potentially prompting hair regrowth.

Biologic Drugs: Some individuals with more severe or widespread alopecia areata might be prescribed biologic drugs like Janus kinase (JAK) inhibitors. These drugs target specific immune pathways involved in hair loss and have shown promise in promoting hair regrowth in clinical trials.

Light Therapy: Phototherapy, involving exposure to ultraviolet light under medical supervision, is another option that may stimulate hair growth in some cases.

Hair Transplantation: For individuals with extensive hair loss and stable disease, hair transplantation techniques might be considered to transplant healthy hair follicles to bald areas.

The choice of treatment depends on various factors, including the extent of hair loss, the patient's age, overall health, and personal preferences. A dermatologist assesses these factors to tailor a treatment plan that suits the individual's needs.

AYURVEDIC TREATMENT OF ALOPECIA AREATA

Ayurveda, an ancient holistic healing system from India, offers a comprehensive approach to address various health conditions, including alopecia areata. The treatment in Ayurveda focuses on restoring balance within the body and addressing potential underlying causes of the condition.

Diet and Lifestyle: Ayurveda emphasizes the significance of a balanced diet and lifestyle modifications. Dietary recommendations might include consuming foods that pacify the body's doshas (Vata, Pitta, Kapha), such as fresh fruits, vegetables, whole grains, and herbs, while avoiding excessively spicy or oily foods.

Herbal Remedies: Ayurvedic practitioners often prescribe herbal supplements or formulations to address imbalances in the body. Some commonly used herbs for alopecia areata might include Amla (Indian gooseberry), Bhringraj (Eclipta alba), Brahmi (Bacopa monnieri), Ashwagandha (Withania somnifera), and Neem (Azadirachta indica). These herbs are believed to have properties that nourish the scalp, promote hair growth, and balance doshas.

Ayurvedic Oil Massage: Massaging the scalp with specific herbal oils like coconut oil infused with herbs such as Bhringraj or Brahmi is a common practice. This massage is believed to improve blood circulation to the scalp, nourish hair follicles, and promote hair growth.

Ayurvedic Therapies: Panchakarma, a set of detoxification and rejuvenation therapies in Ayurveda, might be recommended to eliminate toxins from the body and restore balance. These therapies, which include procedures like Shirodhara (oil dripping on the forehead) and Nasya (nasal administration of herbal oils), aim to address imbalances that could contribute to alopecia areata.

Yoga and Meditation: Stress management is crucial in Ayurveda. Practices like yoga, pranayama (breathing exercises), and meditation are recommended to reduce stress levels, which might play a role in triggering or exacerbating alopecia areata.

It's important to note that while Ayurvedic treatments offer holistic approaches, scientific evidence supporting their efficacy in treating alopecia areata is limited. Additionally, individual responses to these treatments may vary, and consulting a qualified Ayurvedic practitioner is essential to receive personalized treatment based on one's unique constitution and condition.

Combining Ayurvedic treatments with conventional medical approaches under the guidance of healthcare professionals could provide a holistic approach to managing alopecia areata, addressing both physical and mental aspects of the condition.

COSMETIC TREATMENT OF ALOPECIA AREATA

Cosmetic treatments play a crucial role in managing the visible effects of alopecia areata, helping individuals cope with the emotional impact of hair loss and boosting their confidence. While these treatments don't address the underlying cause, they focus on concealing or enhancing the appearance of affected areas.

Wigs and Hairpieces: Wigs made from natural or synthetic hair offer a non-invasive way to cover bald patches on the scalp. They come in various styles, colors, and textures, providing individuals the flexibility to choose a look that suits their preferences.

Hair Camouflage Products: Specialized hair fibers, sprays, or powders designed to match natural hair colors can be applied to the scalp to camouflage bald spots temporarily. These products adhere to existing hair strands, creating an illusion of fuller hair and covering the patches of hair loss.

Scalp Micropigmentation (SMP): SMP is a cosmetic procedure that involves tattooing tiny dots on the scalp to mimic the appearance of hair follicles, giving the impression of a closely cropped hairstyle. This technique can be effective in concealing larger areas of hair loss and providing a more defined look to the scalp.

Cosmetic Tattooing: Some individuals opt for permanent makeup techniques like microblading or eyebrow tattooing to recreate the appearance of eyebrows in cases where alopecia areata affects these areas.

Hairstyling and Camouflaging Techniques: Styling hair creatively or using specific haircuts can help minimize the visibility of bald patches. Certain hairstyles, like layered cuts or strategically placed hair, can divert attention from areas of hair loss.

Hair Building Fibers: These are natural keratin fibers statically charged to cling to existing hair, adding density and volume to thinning areas.

Hair Transplantation: Though not purely cosmetic, hair transplantation techniques involve moving hair follicles from areas unaffected by alopecia areata to the bald patches. This surgical procedure can provide a more permanent solution for some individuals.

Cosmetic treatments offer individuals with alopecia areata various options to manage the visible effects of hair loss, providing them with the freedom to choose the solution that best fits their lifestyle, preferences, and comfort level.

CHAPTER 4

LIFESTYLE MANAGEMENT

NUTRITION AND ITS ROLE IN ALOPECIA AREATA

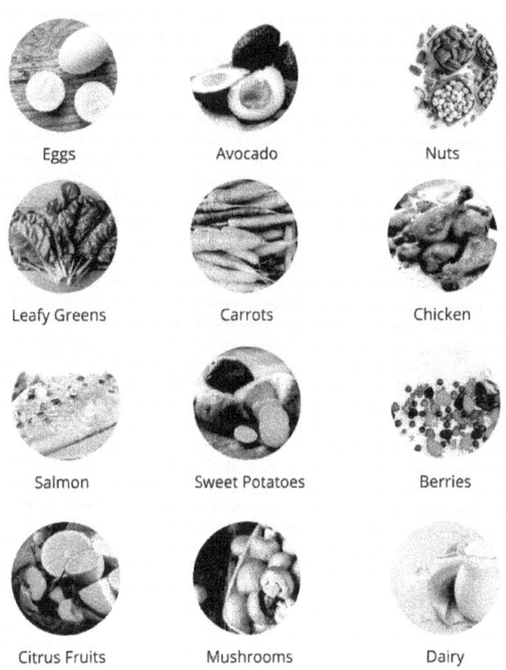

Nutrition plays a pivotal role in maintaining overall health, including the health of our hair. Alopecia areata, a condition characterized by sudden hair loss, can be influenced by various factors, including genetics, autoimmune responses, and nutrient deficiencies. The link between nutrition and alopecia areata underscores the significance of a balanced diet in supporting hair health and potentially managing this condition.

One crucial nutrient for hair health is protein, which comprises the structure of hair strands. A deficiency in protein can lead to weakened hair follicles, resulting in hair loss or thinning. Incorporating sources of lean protein, such as poultry, fish, beans, and nuts, can aid in maintaining hair strength and growth.

Vitamins and minerals also play vital roles. Vitamin D, known for its impact on immune function, has been linked to autoimmune conditions like alopecia areata. Ensuring adequate levels of Vitamin D through sunlight exposure and dietary sources like fortified foods or supplements might help manage its effects.

Similarly, deficiencies in essential minerals like iron, zinc, and biotin have been associated with hair loss. Iron supports the production of red blood cells, which transport oxygen to hair follicles. Zinc contributes to hair tissue growth and repair, while biotin is integral to the production of keratin, a key component of hair structure. Consuming iron-rich foods, such as leafy greens and red meat, along with sources of zinc like nuts and seeds, and biotin from eggs or whole grains, can aid in maintaining healthy hair.

Moreover, omega-3 fatty acids found in fish, flaxseeds, and walnuts have anti-inflammatory properties that may help alleviate some symptoms of alopecia areata, as inflammation is believed to play a role in the condition.

While nutritional adjustments might not be a cure for alopecia areata, they can contribute to overall health and potentially assist in managing the condition. Consulting with healthcare professionals, such as dermatologists or nutritionists, to create a personalized dietary plan, combined with appropriate medical treatment, can offer a holistic approach to addressing alopecia areata and supporting optimal hair health.

HAIRCARE TIPS FOR MANAGING ALOPECIA AREATA

Managing alopecia areata involves both care for existing hair and attention to overall scalp health. Here are some haircare tips that might help:

Gentle Hair Care: Use mild, sulfate-free shampoos and conditioners to avoid further irritation to the scalp. Be gentle while washing and brushing to prevent additional stress on the hair follicles.

Avoid Harsh Styling: Minimize the use of heated styling tools, tight hairstyles (like ponytails or braids), and chemical treatments, as they can weaken the hair and exacerbate the condition.

Scalp Massage: Regular, gentle scalp massages can help stimulate blood flow to the hair follicles, potentially promoting hair growth. Use your fingertips in a circular motion to massage the scalp.

Balanced Diet: Ensure your diet includes a variety of nutrients essential for hair health, such as protein, iron, zinc, biotin, omega-3 fatty acids, and vitamins A, C, and D. A balanced diet can support overall health and potentially aid in managing alopecia areata.

Stress Management: Stress can exacerbate certain health conditions, including alopecia areata. Practice stress-reduction techniques like yoga, meditation, or engaging in hobbies to help manage stress levels.

Consult Professionals: Seek guidance from dermatologists or trichologists who specialize in hair and scalp health. They can recommend specific treatments, such as corticosteroid injections, topical treatments, or immunotherapy, tailored to your condition.

Wigs or Hairpieces: Consider using wigs, hairpieces, or scarves if you're uncomfortable with visible hair loss.

They can also protect the scalp from environmental elements.

Remember, alopecia areata varies from person to person, and what works for one individual may not necessarily work for another. It's crucial to seek personalized advice from healthcare professionals to develop a comprehensive management plan suited to your specific needs.

EXERCISE, STRESS MANAGEMENT AND THEIR EFFECTS ON ALOPECIA AREATA

The relationship between exercise, stress management, and their impact on alopecia areata highlights the interconnectedness of lifestyle factors with this autoimmune condition.

Exercise: Regular physical activity offers numerous health benefits, including improved blood circulation and immune function. While exercise doesn't directly treat alopecia areata, it can positively influence overall health, potentially contributing to better management of the condition. Enhanced circulation may aid in delivering nutrients and oxygen to hair follicles, supporting their health and potentially promoting hair growth. Additionally, exercise can help reduce stress, which is often associated with triggering or worsening autoimmune conditions like alopecia areata.

Stress Management: Stress plays a significant role in the exacerbation of various health conditions, including alopecia areata. Managing stress through techniques like exercise, meditation, yoga, or mindfulness can positively impact the body's response to stressors. High stress levels can trigger or worsen autoimmune responses, potentially leading to more severe symptoms of alopecia areata. Stress management practices can help regulate the body's immune system, reducing the likelihood of flare-ups or worsening of the condition.

The Connection to Alopecia Areata: While exercise itself might not directly influence the development or progression of alopecia areata, its impact on stress reduction and overall well-being can indirectly contribute to managing the condition. Stress management techniques, including regular exercise, can potentially modulate the immune response and decrease inflammation, factors believed to be associated with the onset and progression of alopecia areata.

Conclusion: Incorporating regular exercise into a routine, along with stress management strategies, can aid in supporting overall health, potentially alleviating some symptoms or helping manage the effects of alopecia areata. However, it's essential to note that these lifestyle changes should complement, not replace, medical treatment or advice from healthcare professionals. Individual responses to exercise and stress management vary, so consulting with a healthcare provider is crucial to creating a holistic management plan tailored to one's specific needs.

CHAPTER 5

STORY OF RESILIENCE

Living with Alopecia: A Young Woman's Path to Self-Acceptance

Six years old is a young age to become a patient advocate for a health condition. But Laura Pellicano had no choice. In the summer between kindergarten and the first grade, she lost all of the hair on her head, and then soon after, her eyebrows, eyelashes, and all body hair.

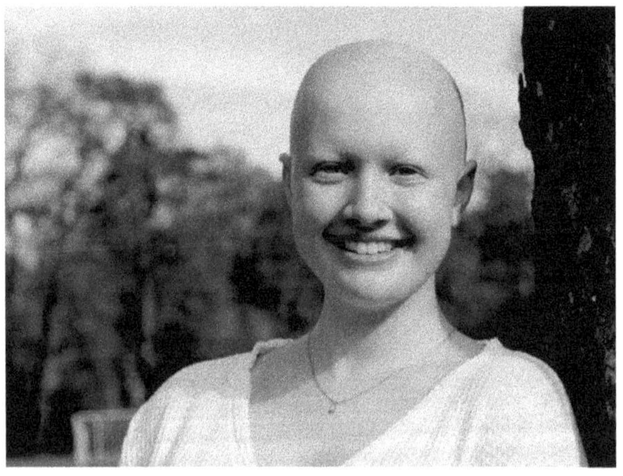

Laura has alopecia universalis, the most advanced form of alopecia areata, a condition that causes hair to fall out on the scalp and/or the body. She dreaded returning to school. "The kids had questions and it's definitely hard being so little and just trying to figure it out. I remember walking in and everyone's like, 'Who's the new girl? Who's that?' And I was like, 'It's just Laura, just me.'"

To help ease the transition, Laura's parents, Debora and Luis Pellicano, helped her prepare a presentation on the condition to give to her classmates that included a Rapunzel-like story of a girl who loses all of her hair. Throughout her school years, Laura, now 19, has presented a similar talk, answering questions about the condition and helping to break stigmas.

People often ask Laura if she has cancer or if she's contagious. She's completely healthy. A sophomore at Northeastern University in Boston, Laura has become a model of self-acceptance, as she's grown up learning to put others at ease with her physical differences.

In some people, the condition can progress to alopecia totalis (complete hair loss on the scalp), and as in Laura's case, alopecia universalis (loss of all body hair). These cases are rare—between 7% and 25% of people with alopecia areata go on to develop the more severe forms.

Researchers are still uncertain of what triggers this autoimmune disorder, although it's believed to be a combination of genetics and environment. About 20% of affected people have family members with alopecia.

A FOCUS ON WELL-BEING

At the age of 5, Laura's parents first noticed her hair falling out while brushing her hair. She was given an initial diagnosis of alopecia areata, but her doctor at the time assured her parents that it would grow back and "it's no big deal," recalls her mom Debora. The family then went through a two-year period of getting a variety of second opinions for their daughter, as well as trying holistic medicine, vitamins and an organic diet. But Laura's hair never grew back.

They reached a turning point when they brought Laura to see a leading dermatologist at Johns Hopkins University, who told them "unfortunately there is nothing you can do to treat the condition," recalls Debora. "Focus on her well-being, on creating a very strong, confident child," Debora recalls the doctor saying. "Keep her busy in different areas, so she doesn't focus on that as much. And don't let this be the center of your family conversation because otherwise, it takes an emotional toll on your child."

For Debora and Luis, it was an emotional adjustment as well. Looking back, Debora says it was hard to even look at photos of their only child, Laura. "My husband and I struggled a lot, especially when Laura lost her eyebrows and eyelashes. For whatever reason, it's such an important definition of her face. The feeling I had was somebody kind of switched my kid right in a matter of a month, because this happened so fast," says Debora, who has served on the board of directors of the National Alopecia Areata Foundation (NAAF) for a decade.

And with her condition so visible to the world, Debora often worried how much it would impact her daughter's life. "The question I had when all of this happened is, 'Is she going to be able to go to college, get a job, be happy and have a normal life?'" says Debora. "There's always that question in the back of my head like: 'Is she okay internally or is she sad?' And every step of her life has always been with this question from a mom's perspective: Would things be easier for her if she didn't have alopecia?"

'THEY LOOK JUST LIKE ME'

With support from her family, Laura found her way and even thrived. Early on, Laura made a choice not to cover up her bald head with a wig or hat. "I just for some reason felt like if I was not going to have hair, I might as well accept it and just learn to live with it and learn to tell people about it," says Laura.

During her elementary school years, she went through a period where she struggled with bullying and constantly having to explain herself to peers. Her parents eventually switched her to a private school, where she fared better in a smaller setting where the kids became comfortable with her.

Connecting with other kids with alopecia has been an important part of her journey. When she was 8, she attended her first NAAF kids camp in Texas. "There were like a hundred kids who looked just like me and I was like, 'Wow, I don't have to explain myself,'" says Laura. Her dad loves telling the story that when he first went to pick her up at the pool, he couldn't locate his daughter in the sea of bald children. "Just having kids that look like you, makes you feel less alone," she adds.

Her NAAF friends continue to play an important role in her life. Although they're spread out around the country, she can quickly reach out to them in their message group to ask advice on issues she's facing.

LOOKING TO THE FUTURE

For Laura's first semester at college, she decided to study abroad in Australia. While any parent would worry about their child being so far away from home, Debora had an added layer of worry of how her daughter would be treated with her condition.

Laura ended up having the best time of her life, she says. "I do remember being like okay this is another time when I have to explain myself. So, I remember one of the first days I had moved in with my roommates and I sat down, I was like, 'Hey, just to let you know I have alopecia and here's some information to read about it.' And they're like, 'Okay that's fine, all right.'" So, I definitely think getting older really helps."

In the future, Laura, who is a biology major, is interested in working in the pharmaceutical industry, and possibly working with patients and clinical trials. "I think that really stems from having alopecia. I've been around it my whole life, so I'm super interested in helping other patients."

Courtesy:
https://www.pfizer.com/news/articles/living_with_alop
ecia_a_young_woman_s_path_to_self_acceptance
Advocacy, Community Involvement and Awareness Initiatives for Alopecia Areata

Advocacy, community involvement, and awareness initiatives play pivotal roles in addressing the challenges faced by individuals with alopecia areata. Alopecia areata, an autoimmune condition causing hair loss, significantly impacts one's emotional and social well-being. Effective advocacy involves multiple facets, aiming to educate, support, and empower both affected individuals and society at large.

Advocacy Efforts: Advocacy for alopecia areata involves lobbying for increased research funding, pushing for legislative support for individuals with the condition, and promoting policies that ensure accessibility to treatment and psychological support. Advocates work tirelessly to raise awareness among policymakers, healthcare providers, and the general public, emphasizing the need for better understanding and resources for those affected.

Community Involvement: Engaging communities is crucial for fostering understanding and support. Support groups, both online and offline, provide safe spaces for individuals to share experiences, seek advice, and offer emotional support. Community involvement also extends to organizing events, fundraisers, and walks to raise funds for research, promote acceptance, and reduce stigma associated with alopecia areata.

Awareness Initiatives: Creating awareness about alopecia areata is fundamental in dispelling misconceptions and fostering empathy. This involves public campaigns through various mediums—social media, workshops, educational seminars, and informational materials distributed in schools and healthcare facilities. These initiatives aim to educate the public about the condition's impact on mental health and the importance of acceptance and support.

The Impact: Collectively, these efforts contribute to a more inclusive society that embraces diversity in appearance and supports individuals affected by alopecia areata. They help in reducing the psychological distress often associated with the condition and pave the way for improved access to treatments and support services.

CHAPTER 6

FUTURE DIRECTIONS

BREAKTHROUGHS IN ALOPECIA AREATA RESEARCH

Breakthroughs in Alopecia Areata research have been pivotal in understanding and treating this autoimmune condition causing hair loss.

In recent years, research has shed light on the complex interplay between genetics, immune system dysfunction, and environmental factors contributing to Alopecia Areata. Significant breakthroughs include the identification of specific genetic markers associated with the condition, providing insight into its hereditary nature.

Advancements in immunology have highlighted the role of the immune system in attacking hair follicles, leading to hair loss. This understanding has paved the way for novel treatments targeting the immune response, such as JAK inhibitors, which have shown promising results in halting hair loss and promoting regrowth in some cases.

Additionally, stem cell research and regenerative medicine have emerged as potential avenues for treating Alopecia Areata. Studies exploring the use of stem cells to regenerate hair follicles offer hope for more effective and long-lasting treatments.

Moreover, the development of precision medicine approaches, including personalized therapies based on an individual's genetic profile and immune system characteristics, holds immense promise for tailored and effective treatments for Alopecia Areata.

The collaborative efforts of researchers, clinicians, and affected individuals have fueled these breakthroughs, offering renewed optimism for improved management and eventual cures for Alopecia Areata.

Promising Treatments on The Horizon for Alopecia Areata

Several promising treatments are on the horizon for Alopecia Areata:

JAK Inhibitors: Drugs like tofacitinib and ruxolitinib have shown promise in clinical trials by targeting the immune system to prevent further hair loss and even stimulate regrowth.

Stem Cell Therapy: Research into regenerative medicine involving stem cells aims to regenerate hair follicles, potentially providing a more permanent solution to hair loss caused by Alopecia Areata.

Biologics: Biologic drugs that target specific immune pathways involved in hair loss are being studied. These medications might offer more targeted and effective treatments.

Topical Immunotherapy: Chemicals like diphenylcyclopropenone (DPCP) or squaric acid dibutyl ester (SADBE) are being explored for their ability to provoke an allergic reaction on the scalp, potentially stimulating hair regrowth.

Gene Therapy: Advancements in gene editing techniques offer the potential for correcting genetic mutations associated with Alopecia Areata, though this field is still in its early stages.

Each of these treatments presents hope for individuals with Alopecia Areata, offering a range of options that might soon revolutionize its management and lead to more effective long-term solutions.

Hope for The Future for Alopecia Areata

The future for Alopecia Areata looks hopeful. Ongoing research, technological advancements, and growing awareness have laid a promising foundation for several reasons:

Advancements in Understanding: Researchers have made significant progress in understanding the underlying causes of Alopecia Areata, especially its genetic and immune system components. This deeper understanding is fundamental in developing targeted therapies.

Innovative Treatments: Emerging treatments like JAK inhibitors, stem cell therapy, and biologics have shown remarkable potential in halting hair loss and even promoting regrowth in some cases. These breakthroughs signify a shift towards more effective and personalized treatment options.

Precision Medicine: Tailoring treatments based on an individual's genetic profile, immune system response, and specific manifestations of Alopecia Areata holds great promise. Personalized approaches could significantly enhance treatment outcomes.

Increased Research Focus: There's a growing interest among researchers and pharmaceutical companies in finding solutions for Alopecia Areata. This attention and investment indicate a positive trend towards developing more effective therapies.

Community Support and Advocacy: Support groups, advocacy organizations, and affected individuals have been instrumental in raising awareness, fostering research, and advocating for better resources and treatments for Alopecia Areata.